Donna Jean's
DISASTER

by
Barbara
Williams

illustrated by
Margot Apple

Albert Whitman & Company   Niles, Illinois

Library of Congress Cataloging-in-Publication Data

Williams, Barbara.
  Donna Jean's disaster.

  Summary: Some of Donna Jean's family are so sure she
will fail in reciting a poem at a school program that
they almost convince her of her inadequacy, until her
uncle's belief in her helps her to try again.
  [1. Stage fright—Fiction. 2. Self-perception—
Fiction. 3. Uncles—Fiction] I. Apple, Margot, ill.
II. Title
PZ7.W65587Do 1986   [Fic]   86-15817
ISBN 0-8075-1682-1 (lib. bdg.)

The text of this book is set in sixteen-point Goudy.

Text © 1986 by Barbara Williams
Illustrations © 1986 by Margot Apple
Published in 1986 by Albert Whitman & Company, Niles, Illinois
Published simultaneously in Canada by General Publishing, Limited, Toronto
Printed in U.S.A. All rights reserved.
10   9   8   7   6   5   4   3   2   1

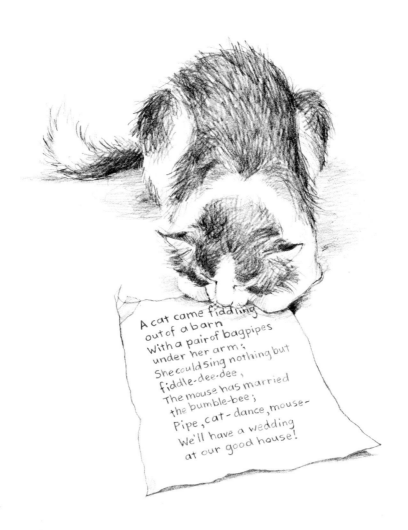

A cat came fiddling
out of a barn
With a pair of bagpipes
under her arm;
She could sing nothing but
fiddle-dee-dee,
The mouse has married
the bumble-bee;
Pipe, cat - dance, mouse—
We'll have a wedding
at our good house!

To John Daniel Williams II :
May he grow up to be proud of his name
and as courageous as his Aunt Kim.

B.W.

On Monday Donna Jean's teacher asked her to learn a poem for the parents' program Friday. The teacher pinned it to her tee shirt, and Donna Jean walked home proudly.

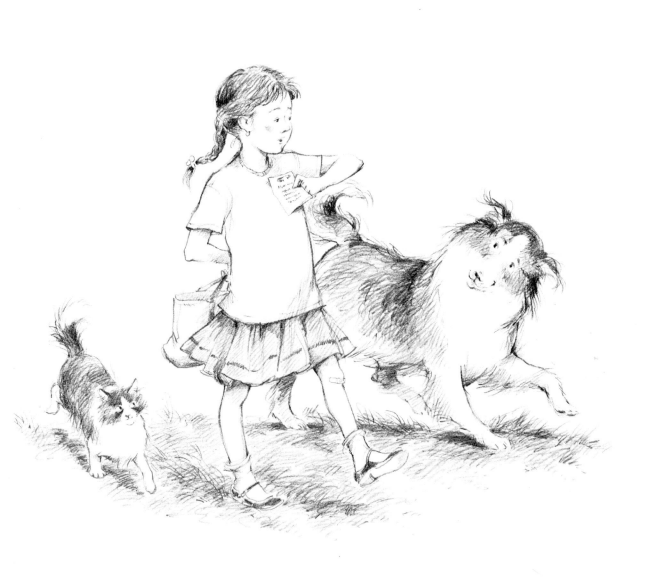

When she got home, Uncle Oscar and her sister, Rosemarie, were on the porch. She showed them the poem.

"Donna Jean can never learn all that!" said Rosemarie.

"Maybe I can't learn all that," said Donna Jean.

"Let's go to the road," said Uncle Oscar. "I want to see if you can still ride a bicycle."

"Of course I can," said Donna Jean.

"Let's go see," said Uncle Oscar.

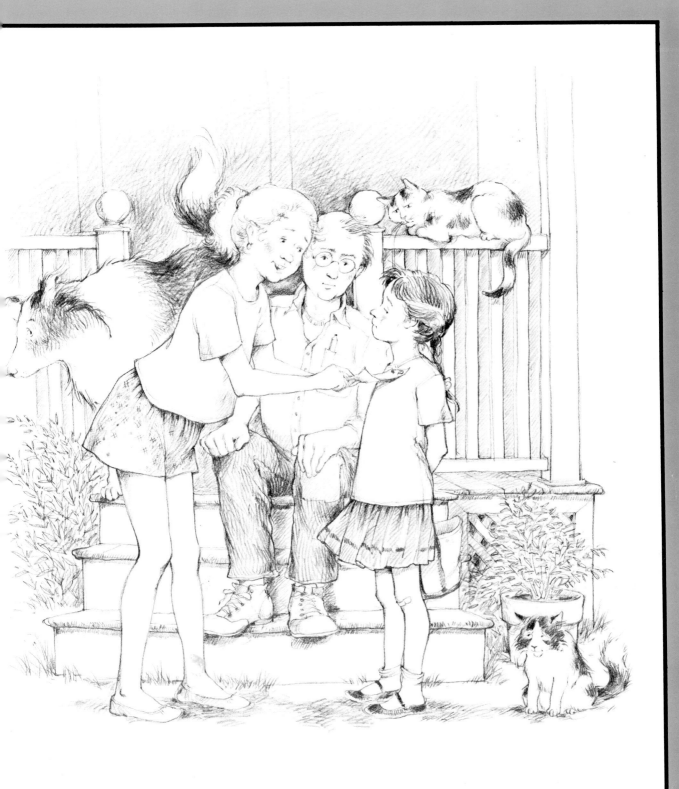

Donna Jean got her bike and rode it up and down the road. "See, I can still ride," she said.

"Remember when you thought you'd never learn to ride? You can do lots of things if you'll just believe in yourself," said Uncle Oscar.

"No one else believes in me," said Donna Jean.

"Of course we do," said Uncle Oscar. "And we'll prove it to you. We'll sit in the front row while you recite your poem and smile at you so you'll know we believe in you."

Uncle Oscar went home to fix his supper. And Donna Jean went back into the house to learn her poem.

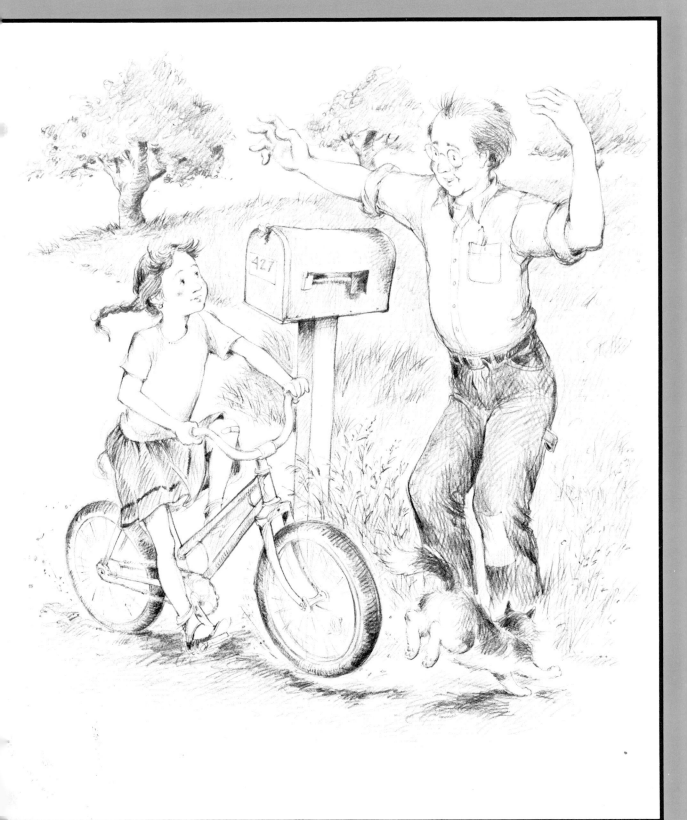

"Let's practice the poem a little at a time," said Donna Jean's mother at supper. "I'll read some words to you and then you say them back: *A cat came fiddling out of a barn with a pair of bagpipes under her arm.*"

"*A cat came diddling out of a barn,*" repeated Donna Jean.

Rosemarie dropped the silverware and howled with laughter.

"No, Donna Jean," said her mother. "The cat was fiddling. That means she was playing a violin."

"You said she was carrying bagpipes," Donna Jean pointed out.

Donna Jean's father spilled the milk he was pouring. "What's the matter with that teacher?" he demanded. "She's given Donna Jean a poem that she doesn't even understand. She can't learn a poem she doesn't understand!"

"Her teacher is trying to embarrass our whole family," complained Rosemarie.

"Maybe I'll embarrass the whole family," said Donna Jean.

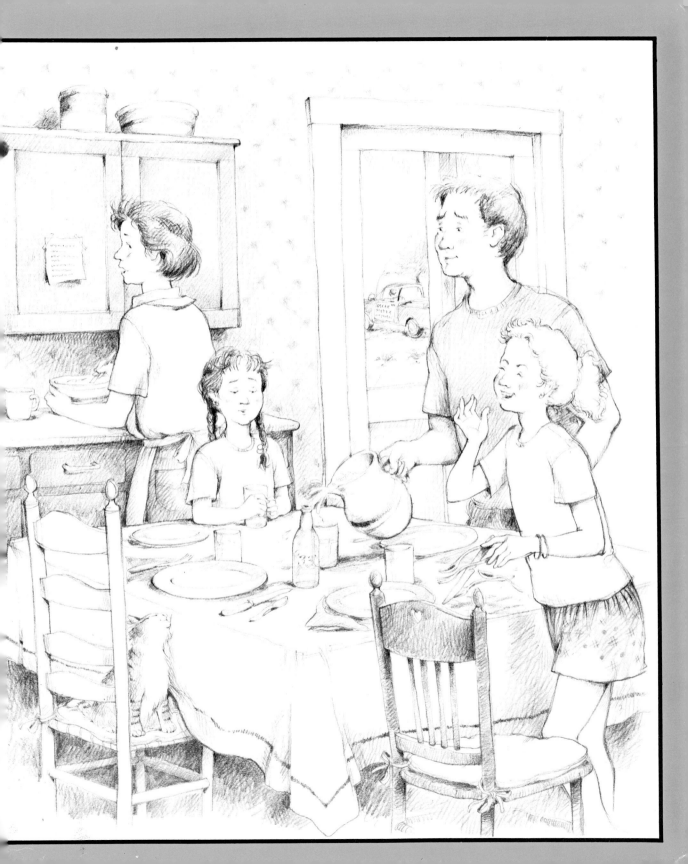

Donna Jean's mother didn't talk much during supper. After the dishes were put away, she tried to help Donna Jean again. She got out an old drum.

"Sometimes the rhythm in a poem is more important than the words," she told Donna Jean. "I'll beat the rhythm as I say the words."

Donna Jean listened carefully. Then they said the words together.

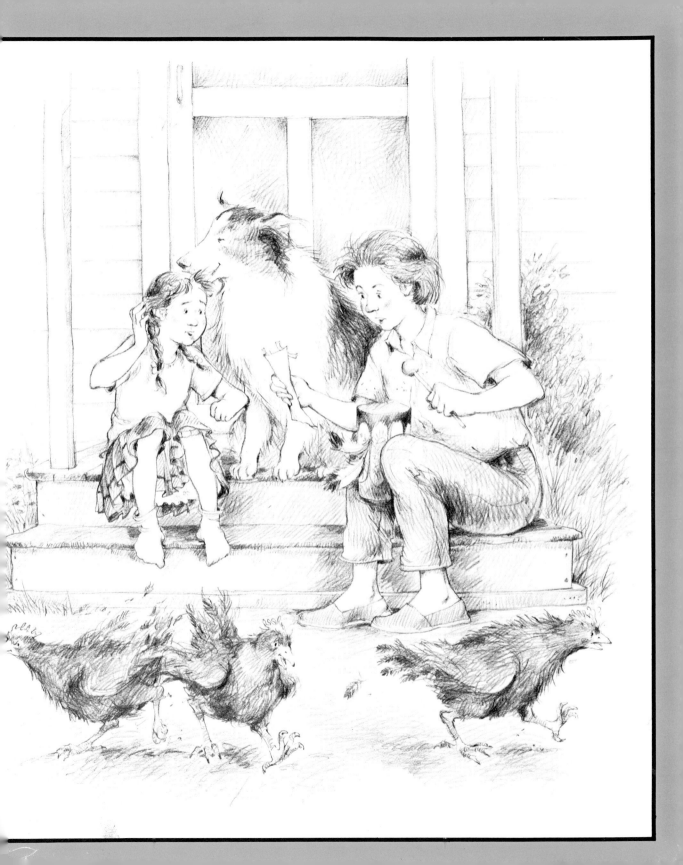

"Listen to Donna Jean!" exclaimed her mother. "She's learned the whole poem."

"Stand up straight and recite your poem, Donna Jean," said her father.

Donna Jean stood up straight and said her poem.

"Isn't that wonderful?" said Donna Jean's mother.

"Nice and loud," agreed Donna Jean's father.

"She talks like a drum," said Rosemarie.

"Hmm," said Donna Jean's father. "Maybe Rosemarie is right. Use your arms more, Donna Jean. Raise your arm when you say 'fiddle-de-dee.'"

"Fiddle-de-dee," said Donna Jean, raising her arm.

"That's better," said Donna Jean's father.

"Yes," said Donna Jean's mother.

"It won't get her a standing ovation," said Rosemarie.

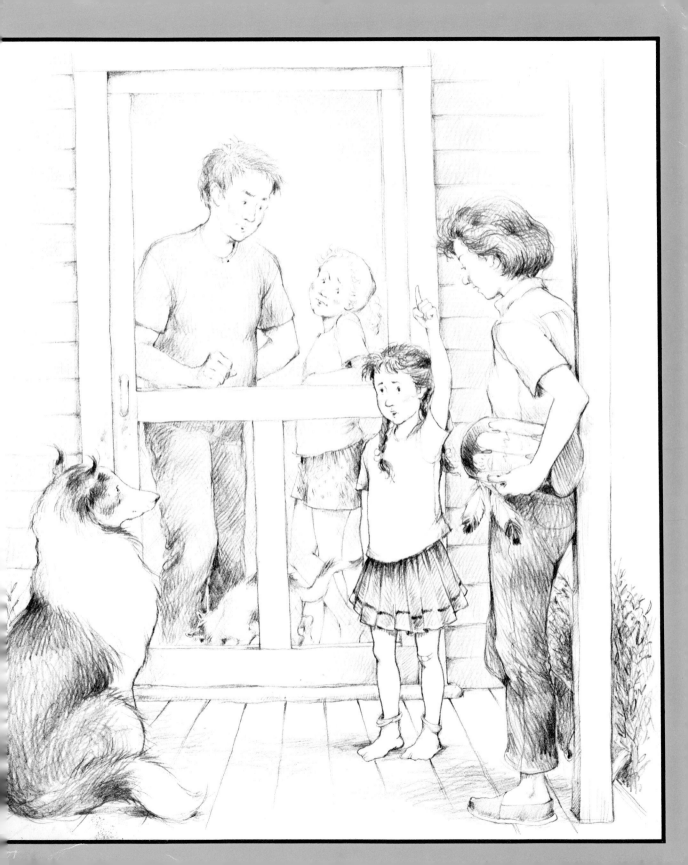

"Don't worry. Not everyone gets a standing ovation," her mother told Donna Jean.

"What's a standing ovation?" asked Donna Jean.

"You'll never need to know," hinted Rosemarie.

"A standing ovation is when the audience stands up to clap for you," said Donna Jean's mother. "It means the people really like you. But it doesn't mean that they DON'T like you if they don't stand up. So don't feel bad if they stay in their seats."

"They may be asleep," suggested Rosemarie.

"I think I'll go to bed," said Donna Jean. She tripped as she started toward the stairs.

"Donna Jean is going to trip when she walks onstage," predicted Rosemarie. "And she'll forget her poem. We'll all be embarrassed. She'll be a disaster."

"Maybe I'll be a disaster," said Donna Jean.

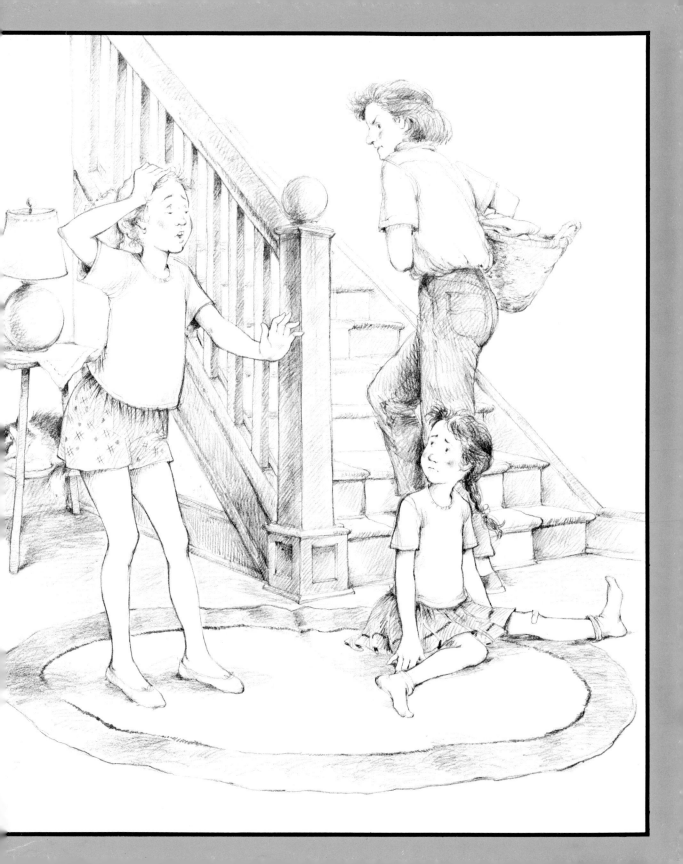

Donna Jean practiced her poem all week. On Friday she and her family got ready to leave home for the parents' program.

"Does Donna Jean have to wear that orange dress?" grumbled Rosemarie.

"I thought she should wear her new plaid skirt," said Donna Jean's mother. "But she wanted to wear the orange dress Uncle Oscar gave her."

"She looks like a pumpkin," said Rosemarie.

"Stop worrying about clothes," said Donna Jean's father. "Let's get going."

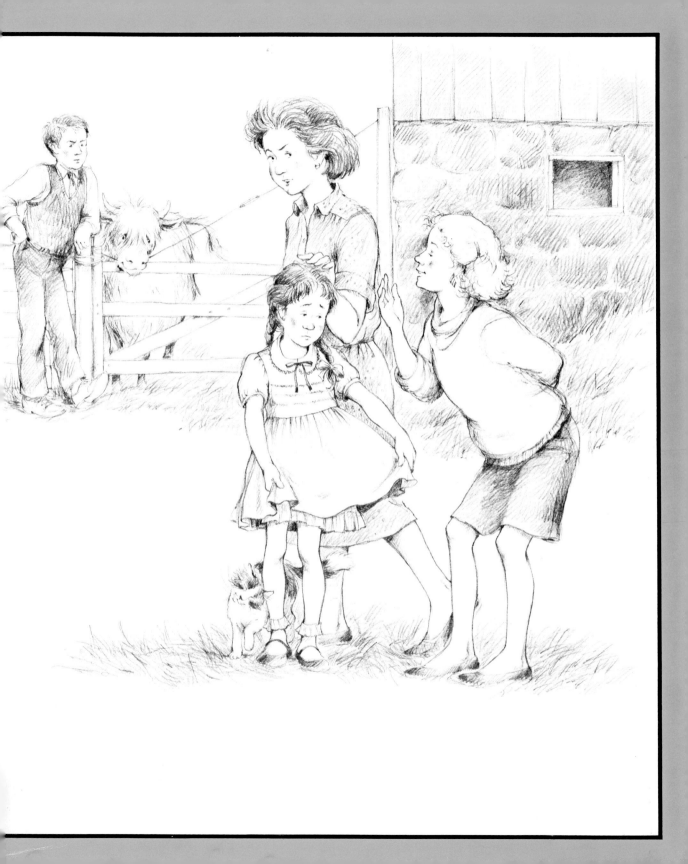

At school Uncle Oscar was nowhere in sight.

"If Oscar comes in late, the ushers won't let him come to the front," said Donna Jean's mother.

"Where is he?" asked Donna Jean. "He promised he'd sit in the front row and smile at me."

"Never mind about Oscar," said Donna Jean's father. "We're here, aren't we? We'll sit in the front row and smile at you."

"I bet he forgot," said Rosemarie.

"Maybe he forgot," said Donna Jean.

"Hurry and go backstage, dear," said Donna Jean's mother. "It's time for the program to start."

Uncle Oscar ran into the auditorium just as the program began, and the usher made him take a seat at the back.

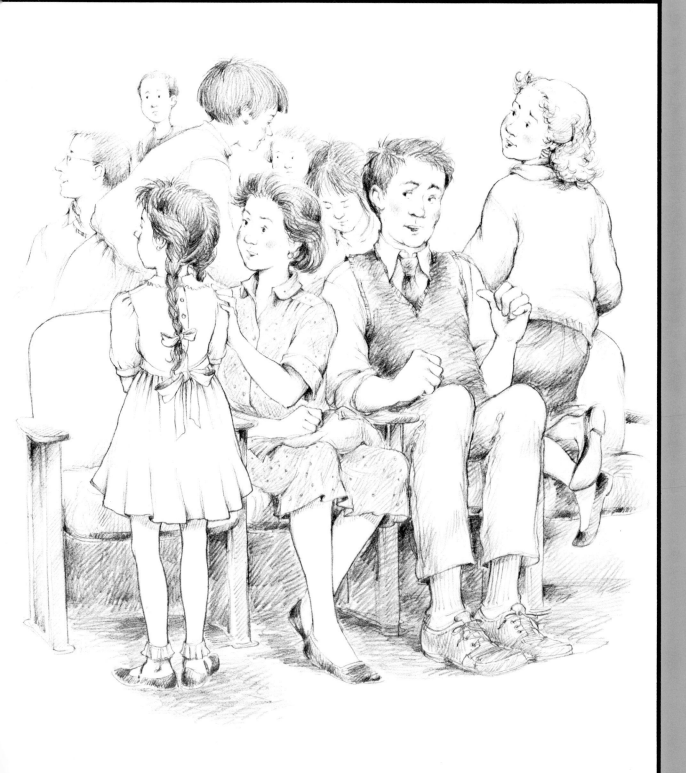

Several children sang together. Then the teacher announced Donna Jean's poem. Donna Jean tripped as she walked onstage, and a few people laughed.

"I told you so," Rosemarie whispered loudly.

Donna Jean looked at Uncle Oscar's empty seat in the front row. Then she looked at the other members of her family. Her mother seemed worried. Her father seemed cross. Rosemarie seemed embarrassed.

"Uh — uh — uh," stammered Donna Jean.

From his seat near the back, Uncle Oscar waved and smiled at Donna Jean, but she didn't see him.

"Uh — uh — uh," said Donna Jean.

"A CAT," called her mother.

"A cat — a cat —" stammered Donna Jean.

More people laughed, so Uncle Oscar waved and smiled harder. But Donna Jean didn't notice.

"A CAT CAME FIDDLING," called Donna Jean's mother anxiously.

"Oooh, she forgot her lines," moaned Rosemarie. "She's really going to mess up."

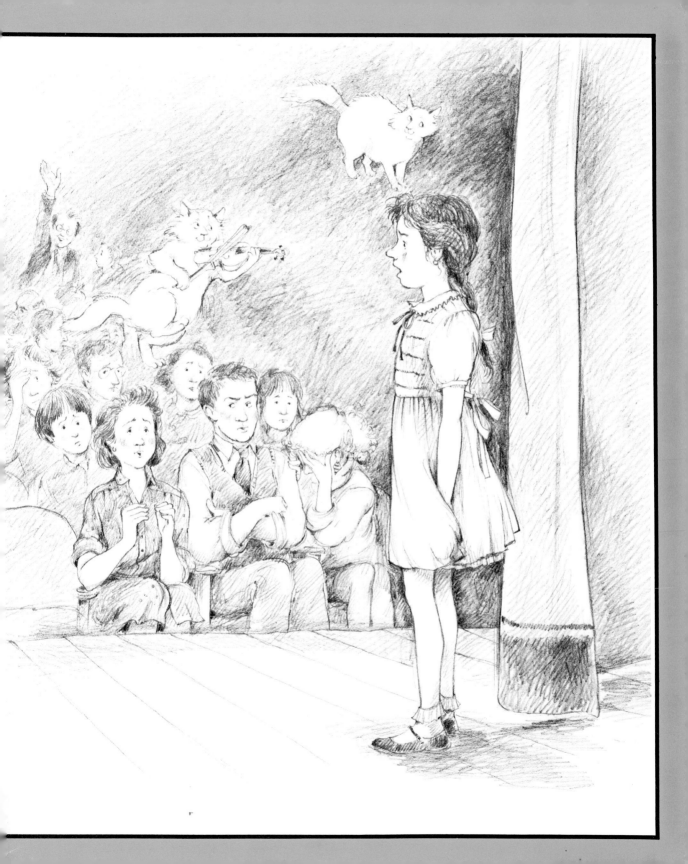

Donna Jean felt dizzy, and she couldn't remember any words of her poem. She ran offstage and into the hall.

Uncle Oscar pushed an usher aside and raced down to the front row.

Rosemarie and her parents hurried out in the hall to find Donna Jean. She was crying into the hem of her orange dress.

Her mother threw her arms around Donna Jean and held her close.

"I embarrassed you all," sobbed Donna Jean. "Rosemarie's right. I'm a disaster."

"It was my fault," said her mother. "I'm sorry I shouted the words at you."

"I can't ever go to school again," said Donna Jean. "I'll never be able to face my friends."

"It's not so bad to look like a pumpkin," said Rosemarie. "Anyway, you just tripped. You didn't fall all the way down."

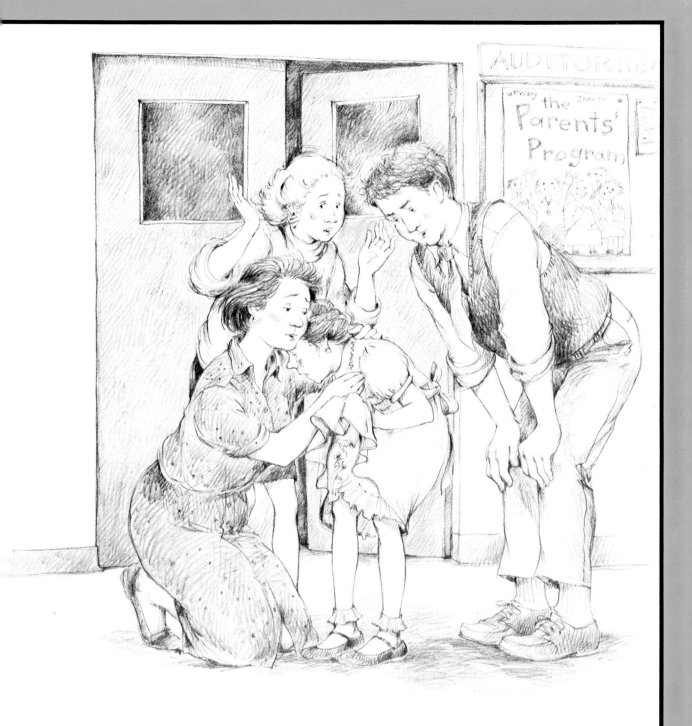

"It was the teacher's fault," said Donna Jean's father. "She shouldn't have given you such a hard poem. It was Oscar's fault, too. He should have come on time."

"He forgot me," wept Donna Jean.

"No, he didn't," said Donna Jean's mother. "He's sitting in the front row."

"With a stupid grin on his face," said Donna Jean's father.

"He says he's going to stay there until you recite your poem," added Rosemarie.

"He is?" said Donna Jean. "Why?" Suddenly she stopped crying and wiped her eyes again on the hem of her orange dress. "OH! Does he really believe I can do it?"

Her mother smiled at her. "Yes, and I know you can, too."

Donna Jean took a deep breath. Then she ran toward the stage as her family went back to their seats in the front row.

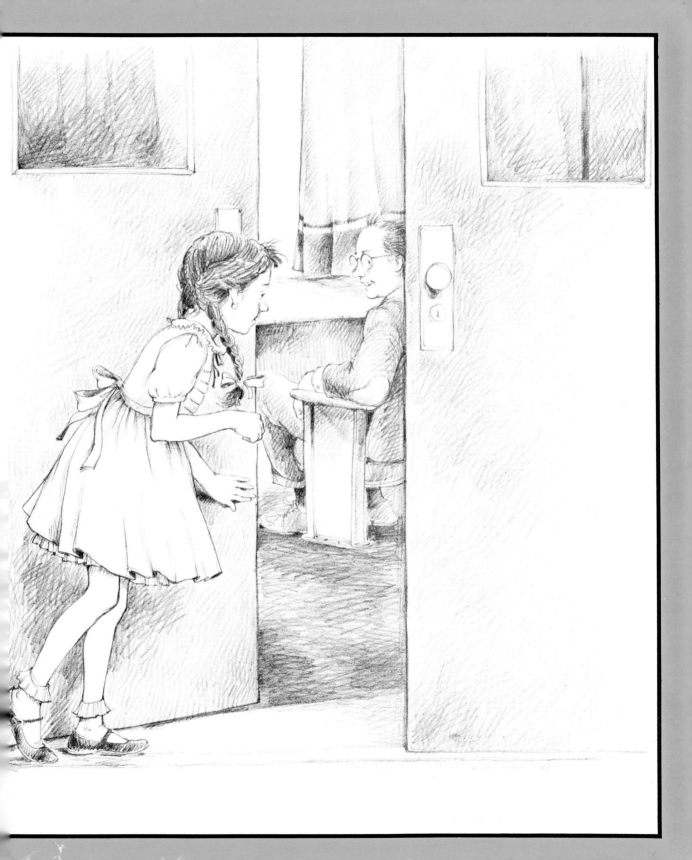

Donna Jean whispered something to her teacher, who nodded. "Donna Jean wants to have another turn," the teacher announced, giving her a big smile. Donna Jean stood up straight and looked at Uncle Oscar. Then she began:

A cat came fiddling out of a barn
with a pair of bagpipes under her arm;
she could sing nothing but fiddle-de-dee,
the mouse has married the bumble-bee;
pipe, cat—dance, mouse—
we'll have a wedding at our good house!

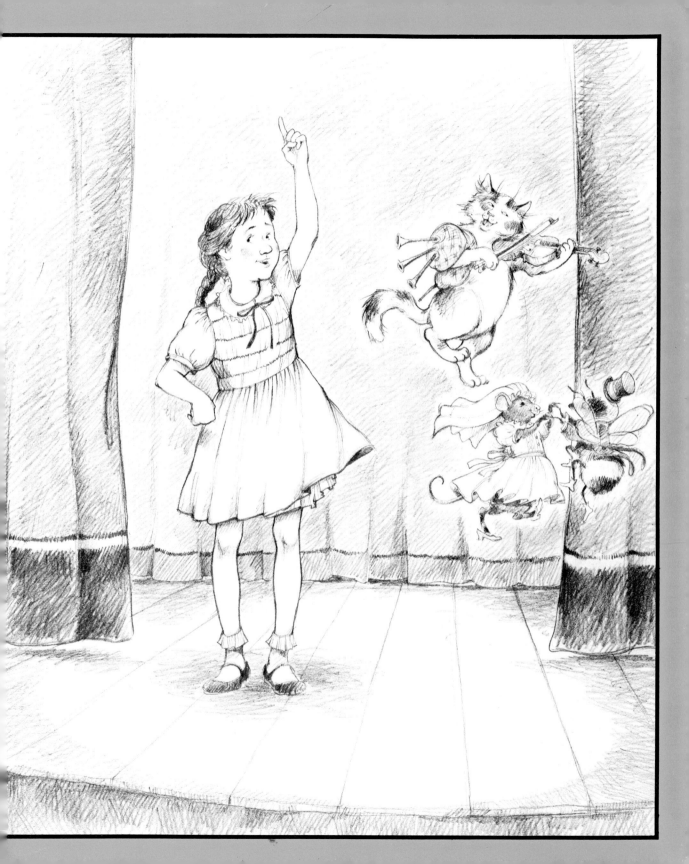

Uncle Oscar stood up, clapping as hard as he was smiling.

Rosemarie looked around and gasped. "Everyone is standing up," she said. "They're giving Donna Jean a standing ovation."

"Of course," said Donna Jean's father.

"She's a very brave girl," said Donna Jean's mother.

"And a very wise girl," said Uncle Oscar.

"She's a disaster," said Rosemarie. "But otherwise she's not too bad."

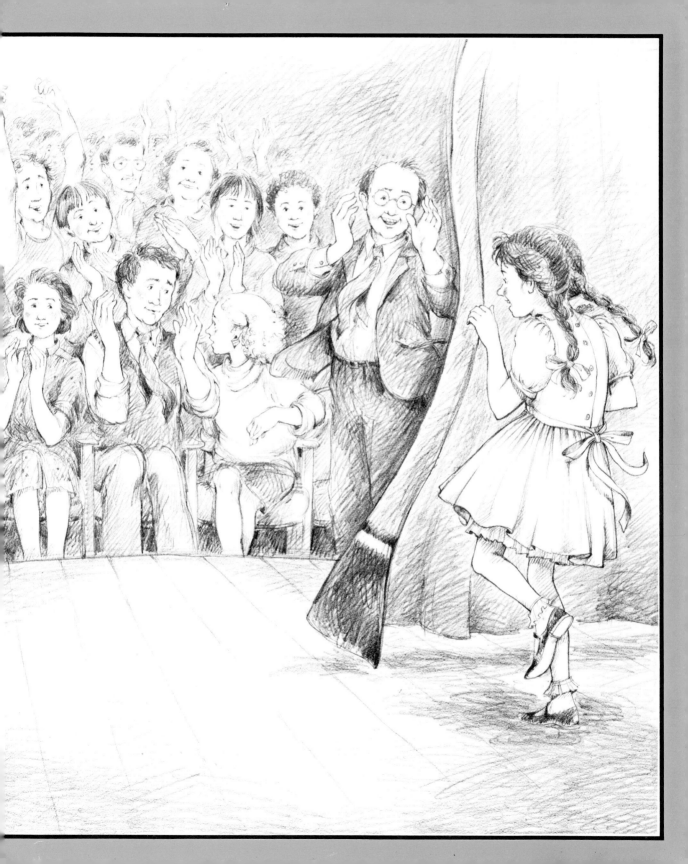

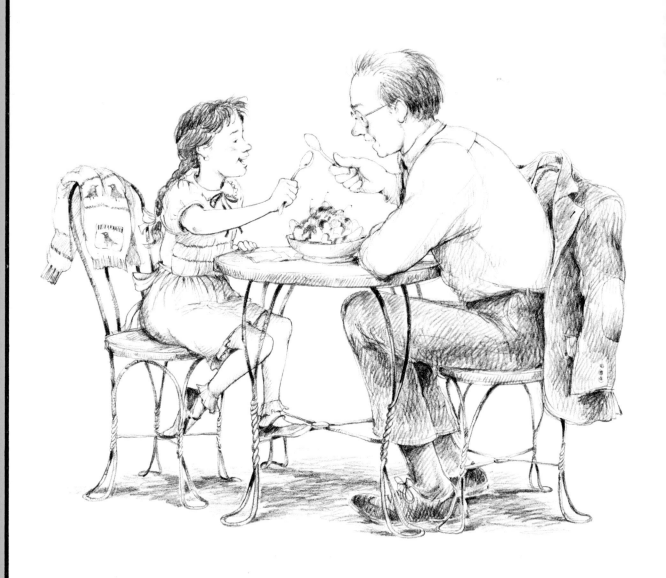